THE BONE HEALTH BOOK

A Complete Guide to Preventing and Treating Osteoporosis

COPYRIGHT

All rights reserved.

TABLE OF CONTENTS

INTRODUCTION 7

PART ONE 10

What is Osteoporosis? 10

Causes of osteoporosis 10

Symptoms of osteoporosis 15

Diagnosis of osteoporosis 17

    1. Clinical Assessment: 17

    2. Bone Density Testing: 18

    3. Laboratory Tests: 18

    4. Fracture Risk Assessment: 19

Importance of early detection and regular screening of
osteoporosis 20

Treatment options for osteoporosis 23

    1. Medications: 23

    2. Calcium and Vitamin D Supplements: 24

    3. Lifestyle Modifications: 25

    4. Physical Therapy: 25

    5. Surgical Interventions: 25

    6. Hormone Replacement Therapy (HRT): 26

    7. Fall Prevention Programs: 26

Prevention of osteoporosis... 27

PART TWO 32

BREAKFAST RECIPES 32

Greek yogurt parfait 32

Oatmeal with Almonds and Dried Fruits 33

Spinach and Feta Omelette 35

Whole Grain Waffles with Greek Yogurt and Berries 38

Cottage Cheese Pancakes 40

Veggie Breakfast Burrito 43

Salmon and Cream Cheese Bagel 45

Tofu Scramble 47

Overnight Chia Pudding 50

Quinoa Breakfast Bowl 52

Peanut Butter Banana Smoothie 55

Avocado Toast with Egg 57

Whole Grain Cereal with Fortified Milk 58

Broccoli and Cheese Omelette 60

Berry and Spinach Smoothie 62

Almond Butter and Banana Sandwich 64

Muesli with Milk and Nuts 66

Ricotta and Berry Stuffed French Toast 68

Brown Rice Pudding 71

Sweet Potato and Black Bean Breakfast Burrito 73

LUNCH RECIPES............76

Spinach and Mushroom Stuffed Chicken Breast............76

Lentil and Vegetable Stir-Fry............77

Greek Quinoa Salad with Grilled Chicken............79

Roasted Veggie and Hummus Wrap............80

Baked Salmon with Quinoa and Steamed Broccoli............81

Turkey and Spinach Salad with Citrus Vinaigrette............82

Chickpea and Vegetable Curry............84

Greek Yogurt and Berry Salad............85

Lentil and Spinach Salad............86

Turkey and Vegetable Quinoa Bowl............87

Quinoa and Spinach Stuffed Peppers............88

Grilled Chicken and Broccoli Salad............90

Lentil and Vegetable Soup............91

Tuna and White Bean Salad............92

Sweet Potato and Lentil Bowl............94

Spinach and Salmon Salad............95

Greek Chickpea Salad............96

Turkey and Avocado Wrap............97

Broccoli and Quinoa Salad............98

Tomato Basil Quinoa Bowl............99

DINNER RECIPES............101

Baked Salmon with Lemon and Dill............101

Quinoa and Black Bean Stuffed Peppers............102

Chicken and Vegetable Stir-Fry 103

Lentil and Sweet Potato Soup 105

Greek Salad with Grilled Shrimp 107

Baked Chicken and Broccoli Casserole.............................. 108

Spinach and Mushroom Stuffed Chicken.......................... 110

Lentil and Vegetable Curry.. 112

Tofu and Broccoli Stir-Fry 113

Tomato Basil Zucchini Noodles....................................... 115

Mediterranean Chickpea Salad with Grilled Chicken 116

Spinach and White Bean Stuffed Mushrooms................... 118

Baked Cod with Lemon and Herbs 119

Butternut Squash and Chickpea Curry.............................. 120

Grilled Vegetable and Quinoa Salad 122

Tomato Basil Salmon... 123

Quinoa and Kale Stuffed Bell Peppers 125

Greek Lemon Chicken.. 126

Lentil and Spinach Soup 127

Broccoli and Brown Rice Casserole 129

CONCLUSION **131**

INTRODUCTION

Osteoporosis is a disease that thins and weakens the bones. Your bones become fragile and fracture (break) easily, especially the bones in the hip, spine, and wrist. In the United States, millions of people either already have osteoporosis or are at high risk due to low bone mass. Osteoporosis, a term derived from the Greek words "osteo" (meaning bone) and "porosis" (meaning porous), is a stealthy adversary that creeps into our lives, gradually eroding the structural integrity of our bones. In essence, it is a condition where bones become fragile and porous, more akin to lace than the robust, mineral-rich scaffold they are meant to be. These weakened bones are less equipped to bear the burdens of our physicality, rendering them vulnerable to fractures, even from the most innocuous of movements. But osteoporosis is not just a matter of brittle bones; it is a silent undercurrent that weakens our very foundation. Beyond the fractures it inflicts, it alters the course of lives, instilling fear, pain, and limitations that ripple through the fabric of our existence.

In the intricate symphony of life, our bones play the role of a silent yet indispensable orchestra, providing the structure and support that enable us to stand tall, move gracefully, and face the demands of daily existence. Yet, beneath the veneer of solidity lies a complex and fragile world—a world where the health of our skeletal framework is determined by a delicate balance of creation and destruction, of resilience and vulnerability. This world is the realm of osteoporosis.

Our journey into the world of osteoporosis starts with a fundamental question: What exactly is this condition? In essence, osteoporosis is a medical condition characterized by a decrease in bone mass and density, resulting in bones that are more fragile and susceptible to fractures. It is a disease that does not announce itself with grand gestures or dramatic symptoms but instead operates in the shadows, often escaping detection until a fracture occurs.

One of the most confounding aspects of osteoporosis is its ability to remain largely asymptomatic until a fracture occurs. It is a condition that thrives in silence, progressing undetected until a seemingly innocuous movement leads to a fractured hip, a collapsed vertebra, or a broken wrist. Vertebral fractures may manifest as chronic back pain and a gradual loss of height. In the shadow of this silent advance lies a critical challenge: early detection and intervention. The absence of symptoms should not deceive us into complacency, for the insidious effects of osteoporosis can be mitigated and its course altered with timely intervention.

PART ONE

WHAT IS OSTEOPOROSIS?

Osteoporosis is a common bone disease characterized by weakened bones that are more prone to fractures or breaks. The word "osteoporosis" literally means "porous bone," and it reflects the condition's primary feature: a loss of bone density and quality. In individuals with osteoporosis, the bone's microarchitecture becomes fragile, leading to increased susceptibility to fractures, especially in the hip, spine, and wrist.

CAUSES OF OSTEOPOROSIS

Osteoporosis is a condition characterized by weakened bones that are more prone to fractures or breaks. Several factors can contribute to the development of osteoporosis. Here are the primary causes:

1. Aging: The natural aging process is one of the most significant causes of osteoporosis. As people get older, bone density naturally decreases, and bone remodeling becomes less

efficient. This age-related bone loss is more pronounced in women after menopause due to hormonal changes.

2. Hormonal Changes:

• Menopause: In women, the reduction in estrogen levels during menopause accelerates bone loss. Estrogen plays a crucial role in maintaining bone density.

• Low Testosterone: In men, low testosterone levels can also contribute to bone loss.

3. Nutritional Factors:

• Low Calcium Intake: Inadequate dietary calcium can hinder bone formation. Calcium is a crucial mineral for building strong bones.

• Vitamin D Deficiency: Vitamin D is essential for calcium absorption. A deficiency can lead to weakened bones.

• Malnutrition: Poor overall nutrition can impair bone health.

4. Medications:

• Corticosteroids: Long-term use of corticosteroid medications (e.g., prednisone) can lead to bone loss. These medications are often prescribed for conditions like asthma, arthritis, and autoimmune diseases.

• Certain Anticonvulsants: Some anticonvulsant drugs used to treat epilepsy can interfere with calcium absorption and affect bone health.

5. Medical Conditions:

• Rheumatoid Arthritis: Inflammatory conditions like rheumatoid arthritis can lead to bone loss due to chronic inflammation and the use of medications that affect bone metabolism.

• Gastrointestinal Disorders: Conditions that affect nutrient absorption, such as celiac disease, Crohn's disease, and gastric bypass surgery, can impact bone health.

• Endocrine Disorders: Conditions like hyperthyroidism (an overactive thyroid) and hyperparathyroidism (overactivity of the parathyroid glands) can disrupt bone metabolism.

6. Family History: A family history of osteoporosis or fractures can increase an individual's risk. Genetic factors can influence bone density and susceptibility to bone diseases.

7. Race/Ethnicity: While osteoporosis can affect people of all races, studies have shown that Caucasians and Asians, especially postmenopausal women, may be at slightly higher risk.

8. Body Weight: Being underweight or having a small body frame can increase the risk of osteoporosis. Individuals with less muscle mass and lower body weight may have less bone mass.

9. Dietary Habits:

• Excessive Caffeine and Soda: High consumption of caffeine or soda may negatively impact bone density.

• High Salt Intake: A diet high in salt can lead to calcium loss through urine.

10. Physical Activity: Lack of weight-bearing exercise can weaken bones. Regular physical activity, particularly weight-

bearing and resistance exercises, helps stimulate bone remodeling and growth.

11. Smoking: Smoking has been linked to decreased bone density and an increased risk of fractures. It may also affect the absorption of calcium.

12. Alcohol Consumption: Excessive alcohol intake can negatively affect bone health. It can interfere with the body's ability to absorb calcium and affect bone remodeling.

Understanding the causes of osteoporosis is essential for both prevention and management. By addressing modifiable risk factors and adopting a bone-healthy lifestyle, individuals can reduce their risk of developing osteoporosis and minimize the potential for fractures and bone-related complications. If you suspect you may be at risk or are experiencing symptoms of osteoporosis, consult with a healthcare provider for evaluation and appropriate guidance. Early intervention and management are key to maintaining bone health.

SYMPTOMS OF OSTEOPOROSIS

Osteoporosis is often referred to as a "silent disease" because it typically progresses without noticeable symptoms until a fracture occurs. Here are the primary symptoms and signs of osteoporosis:

• Fractures: Fragility fractures are a hallmark of osteoporosis. These fractures occur with minimal or no trauma, often during routine activities or minor falls. Common fracture sites include:

• Hip: Hip fractures are particularly serious and often require surgery. They can lead to mobility issues and increased mortality, especially in older adults.

• Spine: Vertebral fractures, also known as compression fractures, can cause severe back pain and lead to a loss of height and a stooped posture (kyphosis). Multiple vertebral fractures can significantly impact spinal alignment.

• Wrist: Fractures of the wrist bones (typically the distal radius) can occur with a fall on an outstretched hand.

• Back Pain: Vertebral fractures may manifest as chronic back pain. This pain can range from mild discomfort to severe, depending on the extent of the fracture. The pain is often described as deep and aching, and it may worsen with movement or standing.

• Loss of Height: Over time, as vertebral fractures accumulate, individuals with osteoporosis may experience a gradual loss of height. This height loss is primarily due to the compression of vertebral bodies and the resulting changes in spinal alignment.

• Change in Posture: Multiple vertebral fractures can lead to a stooped or hunched posture, known as kyphosis or "dowager's hump." This change in posture is more common in older adults with advanced osteoporosis.

It's essential to recognize that the absence of symptoms does not rule out the presence of osteoporosis. Osteoporosis often remains asymptomatic until a fracture occurs. Therefore, early detection through bone density testing is crucial, especially for individuals with risk factors, those in older age groups, or postmenopausal women. Diagnosing osteoporosis in its early stages allows for appropriate intervention and management to prevent fractures and minimize the impact of the disease on bone health. If you suspect you may be at risk or are experiencing symptoms of osteoporosis, consult with a healthcare provider for evaluation and guidance.

DIAGNOSIS OF OSTEOPOROSIS

Diagnosing osteoporosis typically involves a combination of medical assessments, imaging studies, and laboratory tests. The primary tools and methods used for diagnosing osteoporosis are:

1. Clinical Assessment:

• Medical History: Your healthcare provider will start by taking a detailed medical history. They will inquire about risk factors, such as family history of osteoporosis, any previous fractures, medication use, hormonal history (including menopause), and lifestyle factors (e.g., diet, exercise, smoking, alcohol consumption).

• Physical Examination: During a physical examination, your healthcare provider may assess your posture, height, and mobility. They may also look for signs of fractures or spinal deformities.

2. Bone Density Testing:

• Dual-Energy X-ray Absorptiometry (DXA or DEXA): This is the most common and widely used test for diagnosing osteoporosis. It measures bone mineral density (BMD) at various sites, such as the hip, spine, and sometimes the wrist. DXA results are reported as T-scores and Z-scores:

• T-score: Compares your BMD to that of a healthy young adult of the same gender. A T-score of -1.0 or higher is considered normal, while a T-score of -2.5 or lower indicates osteoporosis.

• Z-score: Compares your BMD to that of individuals of the same age, gender, and ethnicity. A lower Z-score may suggest lower-than-expected bone density for your age group.

3. Laboratory Tests:

• Blood Tests: Blood tests may be conducted to rule out other medical conditions that can affect bone health. These tests may include measurements of calcium, vitamin D, thyroid hormones, parathyroid hormone, and other markers of bone metabolism.

4. Fracture Risk Assessment:

• FRAX Assessment: The Fracture Risk Assessment Tool (FRAX) is a calculator that estimates a person's 10-year risk of major osteoporotic fractures (e.g., hip, spine, forearm). It takes into account clinical risk factors, including age, sex, prior fractures, family history, and other medical conditions. FRAX can help guide decisions about treatment and the need for bone density testing.

• Vertebral Imaging: In some cases, imaging studies like X-rays or CT scans may be used to identify vertebral fractures or assess spinal deformities.

It's important to note that the diagnosis of osteoporosis is typically based on bone density test results, especially the T-score from a DXA scan. However, other clinical factors and risk assessments are also considered in the overall evaluation.

If you are at risk for osteoporosis or experiencing symptoms, it's essential to consult with a healthcare provider for a comprehensive evaluation. Early diagnosis and intervention can help prevent fractures, manage the condition effectively, and reduce the risk of further bone loss. Additionally, your healthcare provider can tailor treatment and preventive measures based on your specific diagnosis and risk profile.

IMPORTANCE OF EARLY DETECTION AND REGULAR SCREENING OF OSTEOPOROSIS

Early detection and regular screening for osteoporosis are of paramount importance for several compelling reasons:

• Preventing Fractures: Osteoporosis is often asymptomatic until a fracture occurs. By the time symptoms manifest, significant bone loss may have already transpired. Early detection through bone density testing allows for the identification of individuals at risk and those with lower bone density. These individuals can then receive appropriate interventions and guidance to prevent fractures.

• Reducing the Impact of Fractures: Osteoporotic fractures, particularly hip and vertebral fractures, can have devastating consequences. Hip fractures, in particular, are associated with increased mortality, loss of independence, and a higher risk of nursing home admission. Early detection enables the implementation of preventive measures, potentially sparing individuals from the physical, emotional, and economic burdens associated with fractures.

• Tailoring Treatment: Early diagnosis provides healthcare providers with a clearer picture of an individual's bone health and fracture risk. With this information, they can prescribe targeted treatments and lifestyle modifications that are most appropriate for the patient's specific needs. These interventions may include medication, nutritional guidance, exercise recommendations, and fall prevention strategies.

• Improving Quality of Life: Osteoporosis can significantly impact an individual's quality of life. Vertebral fractures can lead to chronic back pain and a loss of height, while hip fractures can result in mobility limitations. Early detection and management can help individuals maintain their physical function and overall well-being.

• Cost Savings: Preventing fractures through early detection and intervention can lead to substantial cost savings for both individuals and healthcare systems. The direct and indirect costs associated with osteoporotic fractures, including medical expenses and lost productivity, are substantial. By identifying and managing osteoporosis early, the healthcare system can reduce the economic burden of the disease.

• Promoting Bone Health Across the Lifespan: Regular screening for osteoporosis encourages awareness of bone health and the importance of lifestyle choices that support it. It encourages individuals to maintain a bone-healthy lifestyle from a young age, emphasizing the consumption of adequate calcium and vitamin D, regular weight-bearing exercise, and avoidance of risk factors such as smoking and excessive alcohol consumption.

• Personalized Care: Regular screening allows for the monitoring of bone health over time. It helps healthcare providers track changes in bone density and fracture risk, enabling them to adapt treatment plans as needed. Personalized care ensures that individuals receive interventions tailored to their evolving bone health status.

In summary, early detection and regular screening of osteoporosis are essential for preventing fractures, reducing the impact of the disease, tailoring treatment, improving quality of life, and realizing cost savings. Promoting bone health and raising awareness through screening can lead to a healthier population and a reduced burden on healthcare systems. Individuals should discuss osteoporosis screening with their healthcare providers, especially if they have risk factors or fall within high-risk age groups, such as postmenopausal women and older adults.

TREATMENT OPTIONS FOR OSTEOPOROSIS

Treatment options for osteoporosis aim to strengthen bones, reduce the risk of fractures, and manage associated symptoms. These treatment approaches can include medications, physical therapy, and, in some cases, surgical interventions. The choice of treatment depends on the severity of osteoporosis, an individual's risk factors, and their overall health. Here are various treatment options:

1. Medications:

• Bisphosphonates: These are the most commonly prescribed medications for osteoporosis. Bisphosphonates, such as alendronate, risedronate, and zoledronic acid, work by slowing down bone resorption (breakdown) and preserving bone density. They are usually taken orally or, in the case of zoledronic acid, given intravenously.

• Selective Estrogen Receptor Modulators (SERMs): Medications like raloxifene can help maintain bone density in postmenopausal women by acting on estrogen receptors in bone tissue.

• Parathyroid Hormone (Teriparatide): Teriparatide is a medication that stimulates bone formation and is prescribed for severe osteoporosis when other treatments are ineffective.

• Monoclonal Antibody (Denosumab): Denosumab is an injectable medication that inhibits bone resorption and is used for osteoporosis treatment.

• Calcitonin: Calcitonin may be used in some cases to help reduce pain associated with vertebral fractures, but it is less commonly prescribed due to limited efficacy.

2. Calcium and Vitamin D Supplements:

• Adequate calcium intake is crucial for bone health. If dietary sources are insufficient, supplements may be recommended.

• Vitamin D helps the body absorb calcium, and vitamin D supplements may be prescribed if blood levels are low.

3. Lifestyle Modifications:

• Diet: A balanced diet with sufficient calcium and vitamin D is essential.

• Exercise: Weight-bearing exercises, such as walking and resistance training, can help strengthen bones.

• Fall Prevention: Reducing the risk of falls can be crucial, especially in older adults. This may include home modifications, balance training, and the use of assistive devices.

4. Physical Therapy:

Physical therapists can provide exercises and strategies to improve balance, posture, and overall physical function, reducing the risk of falls and fractures.

5. Surgical Interventions:

• Vertebroplasty and Kyphoplasty: These procedures are used to treat painful vertebral fractures. Vertebroplasty involves injecting bone cement into fractured vertebrae, while kyphoplasty involves creating space in the vertebra before cement injection.

• Hip Fracture Repair: Surgical repair of hip fractures is essential for regaining mobility and function in individuals who have suffered a hip fracture.

• Spinal Fusion: In cases of severe spinal deformities or instability due to osteoporosis, spinal fusion surgery may be considered to stabilize the spine.

6. Hormone Replacement Therapy (HRT):

In some cases, hormone replacement therapy, which involves estrogen or a combination of estrogen and progestin, may be considered for postmenopausal women. However, the decision to use HRT should be carefully discussed with a healthcare provider, considering the potential risks and benefits.

7. Fall Prevention Programs:

These programs may involve assessing an individual's home environment, providing education on fall prevention strategies, and recommending assistive devices like grab bars and handrails.

It's essential for individuals with osteoporosis to work closely with healthcare providers to develop a comprehensive treatment plan tailored to their specific needs and risk factors. The choice of treatment may change over time, and regular follow-up appointments are critical to monitor bone health and assess the effectiveness of the chosen interventions.

PREVENTION OF OSTEOPOROSIS

Preventing osteoporosis involves adopting a bone-healthy lifestyle and taking steps to minimize risk factors. Here are key strategies for osteoporosis prevention:

1. Dietary Calcium and Vitamin D:

• Adequate Calcium Intake: Ensure you are getting enough dietary calcium, which is essential for strong bones. Good sources of calcium include dairy products, leafy green vegetables, almonds, and fortified foods like cereals and orange juice.

• Vitamin D: Vitamin D is necessary for calcium absorption. Spend time in the sun, consume vitamin D-rich foods (fatty fish like salmon and mackerel, fortified dairy products), or consider vitamin D supplements if your levels are low.

2. Balanced Diet: Maintain a balanced diet rich in fruits, vegetables, lean proteins, and whole grains to provide essential nutrients for bone health.

3. Limit Caffeine and Soda: Excessive consumption of caffeine and soda may negatively impact bone density. Moderation is key.

4. Limit Alcohol and Avoid Smoking: Limit alcohol consumption to a moderate level, as excessive alcohol can weaken bones. Avoid smoking, as it is associated with decreased bone density.

5. Regular Exercise: Engage in weight-bearing and muscle-strengthening exercises. Activities like walking, jogging, dancing, and resistance training help build and maintain bone density. Balance and flexibility exercises, such as yoga and tai chi, can improve stability and reduce the risk of falls.

6. Fall Prevention:

- Modify your home environment to reduce fall hazards. Ensure good lighting, remove tripping hazards, and install handrails and grab bars where necessary.

- Use assistive devices like canes or walkers if needed.

- Wear appropriate footwear with good traction.

- Exercise regularly to improve balance and coordination.

7. Medication Review: Discuss with your healthcare provider the potential impact of medications you are taking on bone health. Some medications, such as corticosteroids, can lead to bone loss.

8. Regular Check-ups: Schedule regular check-ups with your healthcare provider to monitor your bone health and assess your risk factors.

9. Bone Density Testing: If you are at risk or fall within high-risk groups (e.g., postmenopausal women, older adults), consider bone density testing (DXA scan). This can help identify low bone density or osteoporosis early.

10. Hormone Replacement Therapy (HRT): Discuss with your healthcare provider the potential benefits and risks of hormone replacement therapy (HRT), especially for postmenopausal women. HRT can help maintain bone density but may have other considerations.

11. Fall Prevention Programs: Consider participating in fall prevention programs, which may include exercises to improve balance, education on home safety, and recommendations for assistive devices.

12. Healthy Lifestyle Choices:

• Maintain a healthy body weight. Being underweight can increase the risk of osteoporosis.

• Manage chronic medical conditions that may affect bone health, such as thyroid disorders or gastrointestinal conditions.

Osteoporosis prevention is a lifelong commitment to maintaining bone health. It is never too early or too late to adopt bone-healthy habits. Start by assessing your risk factors, making necessary dietary and lifestyle changes, and seeking guidance from healthcare professionals to create a personalized prevention plan. The goal is to build strong bones and reduce the risk of fractures as you age.

PART TWO

BREAKFAST RECIPES

Greek yogurt parfait

Ingredients:

• 1 cup of Greek yogurt (plain or flavored, depending on your preference)

• 1/2 cup of granola (choose a variety with low added sugar)

• 1/2 cup of mixed berries (e.g., strawberries, blueberries, raspberries)

• 1/4 cup of chopped nuts (e.g., almonds, walnuts)

• 1-2 tablespoons of honey (adjust to taste)

• Fresh mint leaves (optional, for garnish)

Instructions:

1. Wash and pat dry the berries. Chop the nuts if they're not already pre-chopped. Measure out the granola, honey, and Greek yogurt.

2. Start by placing a few spoonfuls of Greek yogurt (about 1/4 cup) at the bottom of a clear glass or bowl. This will be your first layer. Add a layer of granola (about 2 tablespoons) on top of the yogurt. This adds crunch and texture.

3. Next, add a layer of mixed berries (about 1/4 cup) on top of the granola. Sprinkle a few chopped nuts (about 1 tablespoon) over the berries.

4. Drizzle a teaspoon or two of honey over the nuts and berries. Adjust the amount of honey to your desired level of sweetness.

5. Repeat the layering process by adding another layer of Greek yogurt, granola, berries, nuts, and honey until the glass or bowl is filled or until you've used all your ingredients. Finish with a drizzle of honey and a garnish of fresh mint leaves if you like.

6. Your Greek yogurt parfait is ready to enjoy. You can serve it immediately with a long spoon to scoop up all the layers.

Oatmeal with Almonds and Dried Fruits

Ingredients:

• 1/2 cup old-fashioned rolled oats

- 1 cup water or milk (dairy or non-dairy like almond milk)

- 2 tablespoons sliced almonds

- 2 tablespoons dried fruits (e.g., raisins, cranberries, apricots, or a mix)

- 1 tablespoon honey or maple syrup (optional, for added sweetness)

- Pinch of salt

- Cinnamon or nutmeg (optional, for added flavor)

Instructions:

1. In a saucepan, combine the oats and water or milk. Add a pinch of salt. Bring the mixture to a boil over medium-high heat, then reduce the heat to low.

2. Simmer the oats, stirring occasionally, for about 5-7 minutes, or until they reach your desired level of thickness and tenderness. If you prefer a creamier texture, you can add more liquid.

3. While the oats are cooking, you can toast the sliced almonds for added flavor and crunch. Place the almonds in a dry skillet over medium heat. Stir frequently and toast until they turn golden brown and fragrant, which usually takes about 2-3 minutes. Be careful not to burn them, as they can quickly go from toasted to burnt.

4. If your dried fruits are large or not pre-chopped, you may want to chop them into smaller pieces for easier mixing into the oatmeal. Once the oats are cooked to your liking, remove the saucepan from the heat.

5. Stir in the toasted almonds and dried fruits. Add honey or maple syrup if you prefer a sweeter taste. If desired, sprinkle a pinch of cinnamon or nutmeg over the top for added flavor.

6. Serve the oatmeal hot in a bowl, and enjoy! Feel free to customize your oatmeal with other toppings like fresh berries, banana slices, or a dollop of Greek yogurt.

Spinach and Feta Omelette

Ingredients:

• 2 large eggs

- 1/2 cup fresh spinach leaves, chopped

- 2 tablespoons crumbled feta cheese

- 1 tablespoon butter or cooking oil

- Salt and pepper to taste

- Optional additions: diced tomatoes, diced red bell peppers, sliced mushrooms, or diced onions for added flavor and nutrition

Instructions:

1. Rinse the spinach leaves thoroughly under cold water and chop them into smaller pieces. You can also use pre-washed and chopped baby spinach for convenience.

2. Crack the eggs into a bowl and whisk them together until the yolks and whites are well combined. You can add a pinch of salt and pepper to taste at this stage.

3. Place a non-stick skillet or omelette pan over medium-high heat and add the butter or cooking oil. Allow it to melt and coat the bottom of the pan evenly.

4. Add the chopped spinach to the pan and sauté it for about 1-2 minutes or until it wilts and becomes tender. If you're using any additional vegetables, you can add them at this stage and cook until they are slightly softened.

5. Pour the whisked eggs into the pan over the sautéed spinach (and any additional vegetables). Allow the eggs to set around the edges.

6. Sprinkle the crumbled feta cheese evenly over one half of the omelette. Once the eggs are mostly set but still slightly runny on top, carefully fold the omelette in half using a spatula. This will encase the spinach and feta filling.

7. Continue cooking for another 1-2 minutes until the eggs are fully set and the cheese begins to melt. If you prefer a slightly runny center, cook for less time; for well-done, cook a bit longer.

8. Slide the spinach and feta omelette onto a plate and serve hot. You can garnish it with extra feta, a sprinkle of pepper, or fresh herbs like parsley if you like.

9. Enjoy your delicious and nutritious spinach and feta omelette as a hearty breakfast or brunch option.

Whole Grain Waffles with Greek Yogurt and Berries

Ingredients:

For the Waffles:

- 1 cup whole wheat flour

- 1/2 cup rolled oats

- 2 tablespoons brown sugar or honey (for sweetness)

- 1 1/2 teaspoons baking powder

- 1/2 teaspoon baking soda

- 1/4 teaspoon salt

- 1 cup buttermilk (or 1 cup milk with 1 tablespoon lemon juice or white vinegar)

- 1/4 cup unsweetened applesauce (for moisture)

- 1 large egg

- 2 tablespoons melted butter or coconut oil (optional)

- 1 teaspoon vanilla extract (optional)

For the Toppings:

• Greek yogurt (plain or flavored, depending on your preference)

• Fresh mixed berries (e.g., strawberries, blueberries, raspberries)

• Honey or maple syrup for drizzling

• Chopped nuts (e.g., almonds, walnuts) for added crunch (optional)

Instructions:

1. Preheat your waffle iron according to the manufacturer's instructions.

2. In a mixing bowl, combine the whole wheat flour, rolled oats, brown sugar (or honey), baking powder, baking soda, and salt. Stir them together until well mixed.

3. In another bowl, whisk together the buttermilk, unsweetened applesauce, egg, melted butter or coconut oil (if using), and vanilla extract (if using). Mix until the wet ingredients are well combined.

4. Pour the wet ingredients into the bowl with the dry ingredients. Stir until just combined. Be careful not to overmix; a few lumps are okay.

5. Lightly grease the waffle iron if needed. Pour the waffle batter onto the preheated waffle iron according to the manufacturer's instructions. Cook until the waffles are golden brown and crisp.

6. Once the waffles are cooked, transfer them to serving plates. Spread a generous dollop of Greek yogurt on top of each waffle. Add a handful of fresh mixed berries on top of the yogurt.

7. Drizzle honey or maple syrup over the berries for added sweetness. If you like, sprinkle chopped nuts over the waffles for extra texture and flavor.

8. Serve your whole grain waffles with Greek yogurt and berries while they're still warm. Enjoy this wholesome and delicious breakfast!

Cottage Cheese Pancakes

Ingredients:

- 1 cup cottage cheese (low-fat or full-fat, as per your preference)

- 4 large eggs

- 1/4 cup all-purpose flour (or whole wheat flour for a healthier option)

- 1/4 teaspoon baking powder

- 1 tablespoon sugar or honey (optional, for sweetness)

- 1/2 teaspoon vanilla extract (optional)

- Pinch of salt

- Cooking oil or butter for the skillet

Instructions:

1. In a blender or food processor, combine the cottage cheese, eggs, flour, baking powder, sugar or honey (if using), vanilla extract (if using), and a pinch of salt. Blend or process until you have a smooth batter. Alternatively, you can mix these ingredients in a bowl using a hand mixer or whisk.

2. Preheat a non-stick skillet or griddle over medium heat. Add a small amount of cooking oil or butter and spread it evenly to prevent sticking.

3. Pour small portions of the pancake batter onto the skillet to form pancakes of your desired size. You can make them small for mini pancakes or larger for traditional-sized pancakes.

4. Cook the pancakes until you see bubbles forming on the surface, which usually takes about 2-3 minutes.

5. Carefully flip the pancakes using a spatula and cook the other side for another 2-3 minutes, or until they are golden brown and cooked through.

6. Continue making pancakes with the remaining batter, adding more oil or butter to the skillet as needed.

7. Serve the cottage cheese pancakes hot. You can garnish them with fresh fruit, a dollop of Greek yogurt, a drizzle of honey or maple syrup, or a sprinkle of powdered sugar, as desired.

8. Enjoy your protein-rich and flavorful cottage cheese pancakes for a satisfying breakfast.

Veggie Breakfast Burrito

Ingredients:

For the Burrito Filling:

• 1/2 cup diced bell peppers (any color)

• 1/2 cup diced onions

• 1/2 cup diced tomatoes

• 1/2 cup sliced mushrooms

• 1/2 cup spinach or kale, chopped

• 1/2 cup cooked black beans (canned or cooked from dry)

• 4 large eggs (or use tofu for a vegan option)

• Salt and pepper to taste

• Olive oil for sautéing

For Assembling:

• 4 large whole wheat or spinach tortillas

• Salsa or hot sauce (optional)

• Shredded cheese (optional, use vegan cheese if preferred)

• Fresh cilantro or parsley for garnish (optional)

Instructions:

1. Dice the bell peppers, onions, tomatoes, and mushrooms. Chop the spinach or kale. Rinse and drain the black beans if using canned.

2. In a large skillet, heat a tablespoon of olive oil over medium heat. Add the diced onions and cook until they become translucent, about 2-3 minutes.

3. Add the diced bell peppers and sliced mushrooms. Sauté until they start to soften, about 3-4 minutes. Stir in the diced tomatoes and cook for an additional 2 minutes. Add the chopped spinach or kale and cook until wilted, about 1-2 minutes.

4. Finally, add the cooked black beans to the skillet and heat them through. Season the vegetable mixture with salt and pepper to taste. Set aside.

5. In a separate bowl, whisk the eggs (or crumble tofu for a vegan option). Season with salt and pepper. In the same skillet you used for the vegetables, add a bit more oil if needed. Pour in the whisked eggs (or crumbled tofu) and scramble them until cooked to your liking. Remove from heat.

6. Lay out the tortillas on a clean surface. Divide the cooked vegetable mixture and scrambled eggs (or tofu) evenly among the tortillas.

7. If desired, sprinkle shredded cheese over the filling for added flavor. Fold in the sides of each tortilla, then roll it up tightly from the bottom to create a burrito shape.

8. Place the veggie breakfast burritos seam-side down on a plate. You can serve them as they are or cut them in half diagonally for easier eating.

9. If you like, garnish your burritos with fresh cilantro or parsley, and serve with salsa or hot sauce on the side.

Salmon and Cream Cheese Bagel

Ingredients:

- 1 bagel (your choice of flavor)

• 2-3 tablespoons cream cheese (plain or flavored, like chive or herb)

• 2-3 slices of smoked salmon

• Thinly sliced red onion (optional)

• Capers (optional)

• Fresh dill sprigs (optional)

• Lemon wedges (optional)

• Salt and black pepper to taste

Instructions:

1. Slice the bagel in half horizontally. Toast it until it reaches your desired level of crispiness. You can use a toaster or oven for this step.

2. Once the bagel is toasted, spread a generous layer of cream cheese on both halves. You can use plain cream cheese or choose a flavored variety for added flavor.

3. Lay the slices of smoked salmon evenly on the bottom half of the bagel. The cream cheese will act as a creamy base for the salmon.

4. If you like, you can add thinly sliced red onion rings, capers, and a sprig or two of fresh dill for extra flavor and garnish.

5. Sprinkle a pinch of salt and a dash of black pepper over the salmon for seasoning. Place the top half of the bagel over the salmon to create a sandwich.

6. Your salmon and cream cheese bagel is ready to serve. You can serve it as a whole sandwich or cut it in half diagonally for a more elegant presentation.

7. If desired, garnish your bagel with additional fresh dill sprigs and serve with lemon wedges on the side. Squeezing a bit of lemon juice over the salmon can enhance the flavors.

8. Enjoy your delicious salmon and cream cheese bagel for breakfast, brunch, or as a satisfying snack.

Tofu Scramble

Ingredients:

- 1 block of firm tofu (about 14 oz)

- 1-2 tablespoons olive oil or cooking oil of your choice

- 1/2 cup diced onions

- 1/2 cup diced bell peppers (any color)

- 1/2 cup diced tomatoes

- 1/2 cup sliced mushrooms

- 1/2 cup spinach or kale, chopped

- 1-2 cloves garlic, minced

- 1/2 teaspoon turmeric powder (for color)

- 1/2 teaspoon cumin powder

- 1/2 teaspoon paprika (smoked or sweet)

- Salt and pepper to taste

- Optional toppings: avocado, diced avocado, hot sauce, nutritional yeast, chopped fresh herbs

Instructions:

1. Remove the tofu from its packaging and drain any excess liquid. Place the tofu block on a clean kitchen towel or paper towels. Press gently to remove more moisture.

2. Crumble the tofu into small, bite-sized pieces using your hands or a fork. Aim for a scrambled egg-like consistency. Set aside.

3. In a large skillet, heat the olive oil over medium heat. Add the diced onions and sauté for 2-3 minutes until they become translucent.

4. Stir in the minced garlic, turmeric powder (for color), cumin powder, and paprika. Sauté for an additional 30 seconds until the spices become fragrant.

5. Add the diced bell peppers, sliced mushrooms, and chopped tomatoes to the skillet. Sauté for 3-4 minutes until the vegetables start to soften.

6. Add the crumbled tofu to the skillet, and gently fold it into the sautéed vegetables. Cook for another 3-4 minutes, allowing the tofu to heat through.

7. Add the chopped spinach or kale to the skillet. Cook for a few more minutes until the greens wilt and the tofu is heated thoroughly. Stir occasionally.

8. Season the tofu scramble with salt and pepper to taste. Taste and adjust the seasonings or spices as needed to suit your preferences.

9. Serve your tofu scramble hot. You can top it with diced avocado, a drizzle of hot sauce, a sprinkle of nutritional yeast for a cheesy flavor (if desired), or chopped fresh herbs like parsley or cilantro.

10. Serve your tofu scramble as a delicious and satisfying breakfast or brunch option.

Overnight Chia Pudding

Ingredients:

• 1/4 cup chia seeds

• 1 cup milk (dairy or non-dairy like almond milk, coconut milk, or soy milk)

- 1-2 tablespoons sweetener of your choice (e.g., honey, maple syrup, agave nectar)

- 1/2 teaspoon vanilla extract (optional)

- Fresh fruits (e.g., berries, sliced banana) for topping

- Nuts (e.g., almonds, walnuts) for topping (optional)

- Unsweetened shredded coconut or cocoa nibs for topping (optional)

Instructions:

1. In a mixing bowl or a jar with a lid, combine the chia seeds and your choice of milk. Stir well to evenly distribute the chia seeds in the liquid.

2. Stir in the sweetener of your choice (e.g., honey, maple syrup) and vanilla extract if you'd like to add extra flavor.

3. Stir the mixture again after a few minutes to prevent clumping, then cover it and refrigerate. It's essential to refrigerate the chia pudding for at least a few hours or, ideally, overnight to allow the chia seeds to absorb the liquid and create a pudding-like consistency.

4. You can check the pudding after an hour or so and give it a good stir to ensure the chia seeds are evenly distributed. This step is optional but can help prevent clumping.

5. Once the chia pudding has thickened to your desired consistency, usually after several hours or overnight, it's ready to serve.

6. Spoon the chia pudding into serving bowls or jars. Top it with fresh fruits like berries or sliced banana, nuts for added crunch, and optional toppings like shredded coconut or cocoa nibs.

7. Feel free to customize your chia pudding with your favorite toppings, spices (e.g., cinnamon), or additional flavorings (e.g., almond extract). You can also layer it with yogurt or granola for added texture.

Quinoa Breakfast Bowl

Ingredients:

For the Quinoa:

• 1 cup quinoa

- 2 cups water

- Pinch of salt

For Assembling:

- Greek yogurt (plain or flavored)

- Fresh mixed berries (e.g., strawberries, blueberries, raspberries)

- Sliced banana

- Nuts and seeds (e.g., almonds, walnuts, chia seeds)

- Honey or maple syrup for drizzling (optional)

- Cinnamon or nutmeg for sprinkling (optional)

Instructions:

1. Rinse the quinoa thoroughly under cold running water to remove any bitterness. In a medium saucepan, combine the rinsed quinoa, water, and a pinch of salt. Bring it to a boil.

2. Reduce the heat to low, cover the saucepan, and let the quinoa simmer for about 15-20 minutes, or until all the water is absorbed and the quinoa is tender. Remove it from heat.

3. Fluff the cooked quinoa with a fork to separate the grains. Let it cool slightly before assembling your breakfast bowl. You can also make the quinoa ahead of time and store it in the refrigerator.

4. In a serving bowl, start with a portion of cooked quinoa as the base.

5. Add a generous dollop of Greek yogurt on top of the quinoa. Greek yogurt adds creaminess and extra protein to your bowl.

6. Layer fresh mixed berries and sliced banana over the yogurt. You can use any combination of berries you like.

7. Sprinkle a handful of nuts and seeds over the top for added crunch, healthy fats, and nutrients. Chopped almonds, walnuts, and chia seeds are great choices.

8. If you prefer a touch of sweetness, drizzle honey or maple syrup over the ingredients. You can adjust the amount to your taste.

9. For extra flavor, sprinkle a pinch of cinnamon or nutmeg over the top. Your quinoa breakfast bowl is ready to serve. Enjoy it as a nutritious and satisfying breakfast or brunch option.

Peanut Butter Banana Smoothie

Ingredients:

• 1 ripe banana

• 2 tablespoons peanut butter (creamy or crunchy, as you prefer)

• 1 cup milk (dairy or non-dairy like almond milk, soy milk, or oat milk)

• 1/2 cup plain Greek yogurt (optional, for added creaminess and protein)

• 1-2 tablespoons honey or maple syrup (optional, for added sweetness)

• 1/2 teaspoon vanilla extract (optional)

• A pinch of salt (optional)

• Ice cubes (optional, for a colder smoothie)

Instructions:

1. Peel the ripe banana and break it into smaller chunks. This makes it easier to blend.

2. Place the banana chunks, peanut butter, milk, Greek yogurt (if using), honey or maple syrup (if using), vanilla extract (if using), and a pinch of salt (if using) into a blender.

3. If you prefer a colder and thicker smoothie, you can add a handful of ice cubes to the blender.

4. Blend all the ingredients until you have a smooth and creamy consistency. This usually takes about 1-2 minutes.

5. Taste the smoothie and adjust the sweetness or thickness as needed. You can add more honey, peanut butter, or milk to suit your preferences. Pour the peanut butter banana smoothie into a glass or to-go cup.

6. For an extra touch, you can garnish your smoothie with a drizzle of peanut butter, banana slices, or a sprinkle of crushed peanuts.

7. Your delicious peanut butter banana smoothie is ready to enjoy. Sip it as a quick and satisfying breakfast or as a tasty snack.

Avocado Toast with Egg

Ingredients:

• 2 slices of whole-grain bread (or your choice of bread)

• 1 ripe avocado

• 2 large eggs

• Salt and black pepper to taste

• Optional toppings: red pepper flakes, hot sauce, sliced cherry tomatoes, feta cheese, or fresh herbs like cilantro or parsley

Instructions:

1. Place the slices of bread in a toaster or on a skillet over medium heat. Toast until they are golden brown and crisp.

2. While the bread is toasting, cut the ripe avocado in half. Remove the pit and scoop the flesh into a bowl. Mash the avocado with a fork until it reaches your desired level of

creaminess. You can add a pinch of salt and black pepper to taste.

3. In a non-stick skillet, heat a bit of cooking oil or butter over medium heat. Crack the eggs into the skillet and cook them to your preferred style (sunny-side-up, over-easy, or scrambled).

4. If you're making sunny-side-up or over-easy eggs, cover the skillet with a lid briefly to help the eggs cook evenly and set the yolks without flipping them.

5. Sprinkle a pinch of salt and black pepper over the eggs for seasoning. Once the bread is toasted, spread the mashed avocado evenly over each slice.

6. Carefully transfer the cooked eggs onto the avocado-covered toast slices. If you like, you can add red pepper flakes, hot sauce, sliced cherry tomatoes, crumbled feta cheese, or fresh herbs for extra flavor and texture.

7. Your avocado toast with egg is ready to serve. Enjoy it as a delicious and wholesome breakfast or brunch.

Whole Grain Cereal with Fortified Milk

Ingredients:

- 1 cup of your favorite whole grain cereal (look for varieties with minimal added sugars and high fiber content)

- 1 cup fortified milk (such as vitamin D-fortified milk)

- Fresh fruits (e.g., sliced bananas, berries) for topping (optional)

- Nuts (e.g., almonds, walnuts) for topping (optional)

- Honey or maple syrup for drizzling (optional)

Instructions:

1. Select your favorite whole grain cereal. Look for options that are low in added sugars and high in fiber for a healthier choice.

2. Measure out 1 cup of the cereal and place it in a cereal bowl. Pour 1 cup of fortified milk over the cereal. Fortified milk typically contains added vitamins and minerals like vitamin D and calcium, which are important for bone health.

3. If you like, top your cereal with fresh fruits like sliced bananas, berries, or any fruits of your choice. This adds natural sweetness, flavor, and extra nutrients.

4. For added crunch and healthy fats, sprinkle a handful of nuts (e.g., almonds, walnuts) over the top of your cereal.

5. If you prefer a touch of sweetness, drizzle a small amount of honey or maple syrup over your cereal. Be mindful of the added sugar content if you're trying to keep it low.

6. Use a spoon to mix everything together gently. The milk will start to soften the cereal, and the flavors will meld.

7. Enjoy your whole grain cereal with fortified milk right away. It's a simple and nutritious breakfast option that provides essential nutrients to start your day.

Broccoli and Cheese Omelette

Ingredients:

• 2 large eggs

• 1/2 cup cooked broccoli florets (steamed or blanched until tender)

• 1/4 cup shredded cheddar cheese (or your favorite cheese)

• 1-2 tablespoons butter or cooking oil

• Salt and black pepper to taste

• Optional toppings: chopped scallions, diced tomatoes, or a dollop of sour cream

Instructions:

1. Steam or blanch the broccoli florets until they are tender but still crisp, about 3-4 minutes. Drain any excess water and set the broccoli aside.

2. Crack the eggs into a bowl and whisk them together until the yolks and whites are well combined. Add a pinch of salt and black pepper to taste.

3. Place a non-stick skillet or omelette pan over medium-low heat and add the butter or cooking oil. Allow it to melt and coat the bottom of the pan evenly.

4. Pour the whisked eggs into the pan. Use a spatula to gently push the eggs from the edges toward the center as they cook, allowing the uncooked eggs to flow to the edges.

5. Once the eggs are mostly set but still slightly runny on top, carefully arrange the cooked broccoli florets on one half of the

omelette. Sprinkle the shredded cheese evenly over the broccoli.

6. Carefully fold the other half of the omelette over the broccoli and cheese using a spatula. This will encase the filling.

7. Continue cooking for another 1-2 minutes until the eggs are fully set and the cheese begins to melt. If you prefer a slightly runny center, cook for less time; for well-done, cook a bit longer.

8. Slide the broccoli and cheese omelette onto a plate. You can garnish it with optional toppings like chopped scallions, diced tomatoes, or a dollop of sour cream if you like.

9. Enjoy your flavorful and hearty broccoli and cheese omelette as a delicious breakfast or brunch option.

Berry and Spinach Smoothie

Ingredients:

• 1 cup fresh or frozen mixed berries (e.g., strawberries, blueberries, raspberries)

• 1 cup fresh spinach leaves

- 1 ripe banana

- 1/2 cup Greek yogurt (plain or flavored)

- 1/2 cup milk (dairy or non-dairy like almond milk, soy milk, or oat milk)

- 1-2 tablespoons honey or maple syrup (optional, for added sweetness)

- Ice cubes (optional, for a colder smoothie)

Instructions:

1. Wash the spinach leaves thoroughly and remove any tough stems. Peel the ripe banana and break it into smaller chunks.

2. In a blender, combine the mixed berries, fresh spinach leaves, banana chunks, Greek yogurt, and milk. If you're using honey or maple syrup for sweetness, add it at this stage.

3. If you prefer a colder and thicker smoothie, you can add a handful of ice cubes to the blender. Blend all the ingredients until you have a smooth and creamy consistency. This usually takes about 1-2 minutes.

4. Taste the smoothie and adjust the sweetness or thickness as needed. You can add more honey or yogurt to make it sweeter or more milk to thin it out.

5. Pour the berry and spinach smoothie into a glass. Your nutritious and delicious smoothie is ready to enjoy. Sip it as a healthy breakfast, snack, or post-workout refreshment.

Almond Butter and Banana Sandwich

Ingredients:

• 2 slices of whole-grain bread (or your preferred bread)

• 2-3 tablespoons almond butter (creamy or crunchy, as you prefer)

• 1 ripe banana

• Honey or maple syrup (optional, for added sweetness)

• A sprinkle of cinnamon (optional)

Instructions:

1. Peel the ripe banana and slice it into thin rounds. You can also mash it slightly with a fork if you prefer a creamier texture.

2. If you like your sandwich with toasted bread, place the slices in a toaster or on a skillet over medium heat. Toast until they are golden brown and crisp.

3. Take one of the toasted (or untoasted) bread slices and spread 1-1.5 tablespoons of almond butter evenly over it. You can adjust the amount to your preference for nuttiness.

4. Arrange the banana slices evenly over the almond butter. You can place them in a single layer or slightly overlap them.

5. If you like your sandwich sweeter, drizzle a small amount of honey or maple syrup over the banana slices. This step is optional and can be adjusted to your taste.

6. For an extra layer of flavor, sprinkle a pinch of cinnamon over the banana slices.

7. Place the second slice of bread on top to create a sandwich.

8. Using a sharp knife, cut the sandwich in half diagonally to make two triangular halves. Your almond butter and banana sandwich is ready to enjoy. It's a satisfying and nutritious snack or breakfast option.

Muesli with Milk and Nuts

Ingredients:

• 1/2 cup muesli (store-bought or homemade)

• 1 cup milk (dairy or non-dairy like almond milk, soy milk, or oat milk)

• 1/4 cup mixed nuts (e.g., almonds, walnuts, pecans), chopped or crushed

• Fresh fruits (e.g., sliced banana, berries) for topping (optional)

• Honey or maple syrup for drizzling (optional)

Instructions:

1. You can use store-bought muesli or make your own by combining rolled oats, dried fruits, and nuts. Ensure that your muesli doesn't have added sugars if you prefer a healthier option.

2. Measure out 1/2 cup of muesli and place it in a cereal bowl.

3. Pour 1 cup of milk (dairy or non-dairy) over the muesli. You can adjust the amount of milk to your desired level of thickness. Some people prefer their muesli with more milk, while others like it thicker.

4. Give the muesli and milk a good stir to combine. This will help the muesli absorb the milk and soften.

5. Allow the muesli to sit for about 5-10 minutes to let the oats and dried fruits absorb the milk and soften. This is known as "soaking."

6. After soaking, add the chopped or crushed mixed nuts to the muesli. Nuts add a crunchy texture and extra protein and healthy fats to your breakfast.

7. If you like, top your muesli with fresh fruits like sliced bananas or berries. This adds natural sweetness and flavor. If you prefer added sweetness, drizzle a small amount of honey or maple syrup over the muesli.

8. Your muesli with milk and nuts is ready to serve. Enjoy your nutritious and satisfying breakfast. Muesli provides a good mix of complex carbohydrates, fiber, protein, and healthy fats,

making it an excellent choice for a healthy and energizing start to your day.

Ricotta and Berry Stuffed French Toast

Ingredients:

For the Filling:

• 1 cup ricotta cheese

• 1/4 cup powdered sugar

• 1 teaspoon vanilla extract

• Zest of one lemon (optional)

• 1 cup mixed berries (e.g., strawberries, blueberries, raspberries)

For the French Toast:

• 4 slices of thick bread (e.g., challah, brioche, French bread)

• 2 large eggs

• 1/2 cup milk (dairy or non-dairy)

- 1/2 teaspoon ground cinnamon

- 1/2 teaspoon vanilla extract

- Butter or cooking oil for frying

- Maple syrup or powdered sugar for topping (optional)

Instructions:

1. In a mixing bowl, combine the ricotta cheese, powdered sugar, vanilla extract, and lemon zest (if using). Mix until well combined.

2. Gently fold in the mixed berries. You can use fresh or thawed frozen berries, depending on your preference and the season. Set the filling aside while you prepare the French toast.

3. In a shallow dish, whisk together the eggs, milk, ground cinnamon, and vanilla extract. This will be the egg mixture for coating the bread.

4. Heat a skillet or griddle over medium-high heat and add a little butter or cooking oil to coat the surface. Take one slice of thick bread and spread a generous portion of the ricotta and

berry filling on it. Top it with another slice of bread to create a sandwich.

5. Dip the stuffed sandwich into the egg mixture, ensuring that both sides are well-coated.

6. Place the stuffed and coated sandwich on the heated skillet or griddle. Cook for 3-4 minutes on each side, or until the French toast is golden brown and the filling is warm and slightly melted. Repeat the process for the remaining slices of bread.

7. Once the stuffed French toast is cooked, remove it from the skillet or griddle. You can cut it in half diagonally or into quarters for serving.

8. Drizzle with maple syrup or sprinkle with powdered sugar if you'd like, although the sweetness from the filling may be sufficient.

9. Serve your ricotta and berry stuffed French toast hot, garnished with extra fresh berries if desired. Enjoy your delicious and indulgent breakfast or brunch!

Brown Rice Pudding

Ingredients:

• 1 cup brown rice (long-grain or short-grain)

• 4 cups milk (dairy or non-dairy like almond milk, coconut milk)

• 1/2 cup granulated sugar (adjust to taste)

• 1/2 teaspoon ground cinnamon (optional)

• 1/4 teaspoon salt

• 1 teaspoon vanilla extract

• 1/2 cup raisins or other dried fruits (optional)

• Ground nutmeg or cinnamon for garnish (optional)

Instructions:

1. Start by rinsing the brown rice under cold running water until the water runs clear. This helps remove excess starch.

2. In a large, heavy-bottomed saucepan, combine the rinsed brown rice, milk, granulated sugar, ground cinnamon (if using), and salt. Stir well to combine.

3. Place the saucepan over medium-high heat and bring the mixture to a simmer while stirring occasionally. Be careful not to let it boil over.

4. Once the mixture starts to simmer, reduce the heat to low to maintain a gentle simmer. Stir occasionally to prevent the rice from sticking to the bottom of the pan.

5. Simmer the rice pudding for about 45-60 minutes, or until the brown rice is tender and cooked through. The pudding will gradually thicken during this time.

6. Stir in the vanilla extract and add raisins or other dried fruits, if using. Continue to simmer for an additional 10-15 minutes, or until the pudding reaches your desired consistency. You can adjust the sweetness by adding more sugar if needed.

7. Once the rice pudding has thickened to your liking, remove it from the heat. You can serve the brown rice pudding warm or chilled, depending on your preference.

8. If desired, sprinkle ground nutmeg or cinnamon on top for garnish just before serving.

9. Spoon the delicious brown rice pudding into serving bowls and enjoy your comforting dessert.

Sweet Potato and Black Bean Breakfast Burrito

Ingredients:

For the Filling:

• 1 large sweet potato, peeled and diced

• 1 can (15 oz) black beans, drained and rinsed

• 1 red bell pepper, diced

• 1 small onion, finely chopped

• 1 teaspoon ground cumin

• 1/2 teaspoon paprika

• Salt and black pepper to taste

• Cooking oil (e.g., olive oil) for sautéing

For Assembling:

- Large tortillas (whole wheat or your preferred type)

- Eggs (scrambled)

- Shredded cheese (e.g., cheddar, Monterey Jack)

- Salsa or hot sauce (optional)

- Fresh cilantro, chopped (optional)

Instructions:

1. In a large skillet, heat a bit of cooking oil over medium heat. Add the diced sweet potato and cook for about 10-15 minutes, stirring occasionally, until they are tender and slightly crispy on the outside. Season with salt and pepper.

2. Add the chopped onion and diced red bell pepper to the skillet with the sweet potatoes. Sauté for an additional 5-7 minutes, or until the vegetables are softened and slightly caramelized.

3. Stir in the drained and rinsed black beans, ground cumin, paprika, and additional salt and black pepper to taste. Cook for

another 2-3 minutes to heat the beans through and allow the flavors to meld. Adjust the seasoning if needed.

4. Heat the tortillas in a dry skillet or microwave them for a few seconds to make them pliable. Place a generous portion of scrambled eggs in the center of each tortilla, leaving some space around the edges. Add a scoop of the sweet potato and black bean filling on top of the eggs.

5. Sprinkle shredded cheese over the filling. The heat from the filling and eggs will help melt the cheese. If you like some extra flavor and heat, you can add salsa or hot sauce to taste. Sprinkle chopped cilantro over the filling if you prefer.

6. Carefully fold the sides of the tortilla over the filling and then roll it up from the bottom to create a burrito. Place the sweet potato and black bean breakfast burrito seam-side down on a plate.

7. Your hearty and delicious breakfast burrito is ready to enjoy. Serve it immediately, and consider pairing it with a side of fresh fruit or avocado slices for a complete breakfast.

Spinach and Mushroom Stuffed Chicken Breast

Ingredients:

- 2 boneless, skinless chicken breasts

- 1 cup fresh spinach leaves

- 1/2 cup sliced mushrooms

- 2 cloves garlic, minced

- 1/4 cup low-sodium chicken broth

- 1/4 cup shredded mozzarella cheese

- Salt and pepper to taste

- Olive oil for cooking

Instructions:

1. Preheat your oven to 375°F (190°C).

2. In a skillet, heat a small amount of olive oil over medium heat. Add minced garlic and sauté for about 1 minute.

3. Add sliced mushrooms and spinach to the skillet. Sauté until the spinach wilts and the mushrooms become tender. Season with salt and pepper.

4. Slice a pocket into each chicken breast, being careful not to cut all the way through.

5. Stuff each chicken breast with the sautéed spinach and mushroom mixture.

6. Heat a bit more olive oil in the skillet and sear both sides of the stuffed chicken breasts until they are lightly browned.

7. Transfer the chicken breasts to a baking dish, pour the chicken broth over them, and sprinkle with shredded mozzarella cheese.

8. Bake in the preheated oven for about 20-25 minutes or until the chicken is cooked through.

9. Serve the stuffed chicken breasts with a side of steamed vegetables.

Lentil and Vegetable Stir-Fry

Ingredients:

- 1 cup cooked green or brown lentils

- 2 cups mixed vegetables (e.g., broccoli, bell peppers, snap peas)

- 2 cloves garlic, minced

- 1/4 cup low-sodium soy sauce

- 1 tablespoon olive oil

- 1 teaspoon sesame oil (optional)

- Cooked brown rice for serving

Instructions:

1. In a large skillet or wok, heat olive oil over medium-high heat.

2. Add minced garlic and sauté for about 30 seconds. Add the mixed vegetables to the skillet and stir-fry for 3-5 minutes until they are tender-crisp. Add the cooked lentils to the skillet and stir to combine.

3. Pour in the low-sodium soy sauce and sesame oil (if using). Stir well to coat the vegetables and lentils evenly.

4. Cook for an additional 2-3 minutes until everything is heated through.

5. Serve the lentil and vegetable stir-fry over cooked brown rice.

Greek Quinoa Salad with Grilled Chicken

Ingredients:

- 2 boneless, skinless chicken breasts

- 1 cup cooked quinoa

- 1 cup cherry tomatoes, halved

- 1 cucumber, diced

- 1/2 cup Kalamata olives, pitted and sliced

- 1/2 cup crumbled feta cheese

- 2 tablespoons olive oil

- 2 tablespoons lemon juice

- 1 teaspoon dried oregano

- Salt and pepper to taste

Instructions:

1. Season the chicken breasts with salt, pepper, and dried oregano.

2. Grill the chicken until it's cooked through, about 6-8 minutes per side. Let it rest for a few minutes before slicing.

3. In a large bowl, combine cooked quinoa, cherry tomatoes, cucumber, Kalamata olives, and crumbled feta cheese.

4. In a small bowl, whisk together olive oil and lemon juice to make the dressing. Season with salt and pepper.

5. Pour the dressing over the quinoa salad and toss to coat.

6. Serve the grilled chicken slices on top of the salad.

Roasted Veggie and Hummus Wrap

Ingredients:

• Whole-grain wraps or tortillas

• 1 cup mixed roasted vegetables (e.g., bell peppers, zucchini, eggplant)

- 1/2 cup hummus

- 1/4 cup chopped fresh parsley

- Sliced cucumber and tomato (optional)

Instructions:

1. Lay out the whole-grain wrap or tortilla. Spread a generous layer of hummus over the wrap. Place the mixed roasted vegetables on top of the hummus.

2. Sprinkle chopped fresh parsley over the veggies. Add slices of cucumber and tomato if desired.

3. Roll up the wrap tightly, tucking in the sides as you go. Slice in half diagonally for easier eating.

Baked Salmon with Quinoa and Steamed Broccoli

Ingredients:

- 2 salmon fillets

- 1 cup cooked quinoa

- Steamed broccoli florets

- Lemon wedges

- Olive oil

- Salt and pepper to taste

Instructions:

1. Preheat your oven to 375°F (190°C).

2. Season the salmon fillets with salt, pepper, and a drizzle of olive oil. Place the salmon fillets on a baking sheet lined with parchment paper.

3. Bake the salmon for about 15-20 minutes or until it flakes easily with a fork. While the salmon is baking, steam the broccoli florets until they are tender-crisp.

4. Serve the baked salmon on a bed of cooked quinoa, accompanied by steamed broccoli. Garnish with lemon wedges for a burst of citrus flavor.

Turkey and Spinach Salad with Citrus Vinaigrette

Ingredients:

For the Salad:

- 2 cups fresh baby spinach leaves

- 4 oz lean turkey breast, sliced

- 1/4 cup sliced almonds

- 1/4 cup dried cranberries

- 1/4 cup crumbled goat cheese (optional)

For the Citrus Vinaigrette:

- Juice of 1 orange

- Juice of 1 lemon

- 2 tablespoons olive oil

- 1 teaspoon honey

- Salt and pepper to taste

Instructions:

1. In a large salad bowl, arrange the fresh baby spinach leaves.

2. Top the spinach with sliced turkey breast, sliced almonds, dried cranberries, and crumbled goat cheese if using.

3. In a separate bowl, whisk together the orange juice, lemon juice, olive oil, honey, salt, and pepper to make the citrus vinaigrette.

4. Drizzle the vinaigrette over the salad just before serving.

Chickpea and Vegetable Curry

Ingredients:

• 1 can (15 oz) chickpeas, drained and rinsed

• 1 cup mixed vegetables (e.g., bell peppers, peas, carrots)

• 1 small onion, finely chopped

• 2 cloves garlic, minced

• 1 can (14 oz) diced tomatoes

• 1 can (14 oz) light coconut milk

• 2 tablespoons curry powder

• 1 tablespoon olive oil

• Salt and pepper to taste

• Cooked brown rice for serving

Instructions:

1. In a large skillet, heat olive oil over medium heat. Add chopped onion and minced garlic. Sauté for 2-3 minutes until fragrant.

2. Stir in the curry powder and cook for an additional minute. Add the mixed vegetables and sauté for another 3-4 minutes.

3. Pour in the diced tomatoes (with their juices), chickpeas, and light coconut milk. Stir well. Bring the mixture to a simmer and let it cook for 15-20 minutes, or until the vegetables are tender and the curry has thickened.

4. Season with salt and pepper to taste. Serve the chickpea and vegetable curry over cooked brown rice.

Greek Yogurt and Berry Salad

Ingredients:

• 1 cup Greek yogurt (plain or flavored)

• 1 cup mixed berries (e.g., strawberries, blueberries, raspberries)

- 2 tablespoons honey or maple syrup (optional)

- 1/4 cup granola

- Fresh mint leaves for garnish (optional)

Instructions:

1. In a serving bowl, scoop out the Greek yogurt. Top the yogurt with mixed berries.

2. Drizzle honey or maple syrup over the berries for added sweetness if desired. Sprinkle granola on top for crunch and texture.

3. Garnish with fresh mint leaves for a burst of freshness.

Lentil and Spinach Salad

Ingredients:

- 1 cup cooked green lentils

- 2 cups fresh spinach leaves

- 1/4 cup diced red onion

- 1/4 cup crumbled feta cheese (optional)

• 2 tablespoons balsamic vinaigrette dressing

• Salt and pepper to taste

Instructions:

1. In a salad bowl, combine cooked green lentils, fresh spinach leaves, and diced red onion.

2. If desired, sprinkle crumbled feta cheese over the salad. Drizzle balsamic vinaigrette dressing over the salad.

3. Season with salt and pepper to taste. Toss the salad to combine all the ingredients.

Turkey and Vegetable Quinoa Bowl

Ingredients:

• 1 cup cooked quinoa

• 4 oz lean turkey breast, cooked and sliced

• 1 cup roasted vegetables (e.g., sweet potatoes, broccoli, cauliflower)

• 1/4 cup hummus

- 2 tablespoons tahini sauce

- Chopped fresh parsley for garnish (optional)

Instructions:

1. In a serving bowl, place cooked quinoa. Arrange slices of cooked turkey breast on top of the quinoa.

2. Add roasted vegetables to the bowl. Drizzle hummus and tahini sauce over the bowl.

3. Garnish with chopped fresh parsley if desired.

Quinoa and Spinach Stuffed Peppers

Ingredients:

- 4 bell peppers, any color

- 1 cup cooked quinoa

- 2 cups fresh spinach, chopped

- 1 cup canned black beans, drained and rinsed

- 1/2 cup diced tomatoes

- 1/2 cup shredded low-fat cheddar cheese

- 1 teaspoon cumin

- 1/2 teaspoon chili powder

- Salt and pepper to taste

- Olive oil for cooking

Instructions:

1. Preheat your oven to 375°F (190°C). Cut the tops off the bell peppers, remove seeds, and rinse them.

2. In a skillet, heat a bit of olive oil over medium heat. Add chopped spinach and cook until wilted.

3. In a large bowl, combine cooked quinoa, sautéed spinach, black beans, diced tomatoes, shredded cheddar cheese, cumin, chili powder, salt, and pepper.

4. Stuff each bell pepper with the quinoa mixture. Place the stuffed peppers in a baking dish and cover with aluminum foil.

5. Bake for about 30-35 minutes, or until the peppers are tender. Serve hot.

Grilled Chicken and Broccoli Salad

Ingredients:

- 2 boneless, skinless chicken breasts

- 4 cups broccoli florets

- 1/4 cup sliced almonds

- 1/4 cup dried cranberries

- 2 cups mixed greens

- 2 tablespoons balsamic vinaigrette dressing

- Olive oil for grilling

- Salt and pepper to taste

Instructions:

1. Preheat your grill to medium-high heat. Season chicken breasts with salt and pepper.

2. Grill the chicken for about 6-8 minutes per side, or until cooked through.

3. In a pot of boiling water, blanch the broccoli florets for 2-3 minutes, then drain and rinse with cold water. In a large salad bowl, combine mixed greens, blanched broccoli, sliced almonds, and dried cranberries.

4. Slice the grilled chicken and add it to the salad. Drizzle balsamic vinaigrette dressing over the salad and toss to combine.

5. Serve immediately.

Lentil and Vegetable Soup

Ingredients:

• 1 cup dried green or brown lentils, rinsed and drained

• 4 cups low-sodium vegetable broth

• 2 cups water

• 1 cup diced carrots

• 1 cup diced celery

• 1 cup diced onion

- 2 cloves garlic, minced

- 1 teaspoon dried thyme

- 1/2 teaspoon paprika

- Salt and pepper to taste

- Olive oil for sautéing

Instructions:

1. In a large pot, heat a bit of olive oil over medium heat.

2. Add diced onions, carrots, and celery. Sauté for about 5 minutes, until softened. Add minced garlic, dried thyme, paprika, salt, and pepper. Sauté for an additional minute.

3. Stir in lentils, vegetable broth, and water. Bring to a boil. Reduce heat, cover, and simmer for about 20-25 minutes, until lentils are tender.

4. Serve hot.

Tuna and White Bean Salad

Ingredients:

- 2 cans (5 oz each) tuna in water, drained

- 1 can (15 oz) white beans (cannellini or navy beans), drained and rinsed

- 1/2 red onion, finely chopped

- 1/2 cup chopped fresh parsley

- Juice of 1 lemon

- 2 tablespoons olive oil

- Salt and pepper to taste

Instructions:

1. In a large bowl, combine drained tuna, white beans, chopped red onion, and chopped fresh parsley.

2. Drizzle olive oil and lemon juice over the salad. Season with salt and pepper.

3. Toss everything together until well combined.

4. Serve chilled.

Sweet Potato and Lentil Bowl

Ingredients:

- 2 cups cooked brown rice

- 2 cups roasted sweet potatoes, cubed

- 1 cup cooked green or brown lentils

- 1 cup steamed broccoli florets

- 1/4 cup chopped walnuts

- 2 tablespoons balsamic vinaigrette dressing

- Salt and pepper to taste

Instructions:

1. In a large bowl, layer cooked brown rice, roasted sweet potatoes, cooked lentils, and steamed broccoli florets.

2. Drizzle balsamic vinaigrette dressing over the bowl. Sprinkle chopped walnuts on top.

3. Season with salt and pepper. Toss gently to combine. Serve warm.

Spinach and Salmon Salad

Ingredients:

• 4 cups fresh spinach leaves

• 1 grilled or baked salmon fillet (4-6 oz), flaked

• 1/4 cup cherry tomatoes, halved

• 1/4 cup sliced cucumbers

• 1/4 cup sliced red onions

• 1 tablespoon olive oil

• 1 tablespoon balsamic vinegar

• Salt and pepper to taste

Instructions:

1. In a large salad bowl, combine fresh spinach leaves, cherry tomatoes, sliced cucumbers, and sliced red onions.

2. Top the salad with the flaked salmon.

3. In a small bowl, whisk together olive oil, balsamic vinegar, salt, and pepper to create the dressing.

4. Drizzle the dressing over the salad, toss gently to coat, and serve.

Greek Chickpea Salad

Ingredients:

- 2 cups cooked chickpeas (canned or cooked from dried)

- 1 cup diced cucumbers

- 1 cup diced tomatoes

- 1/2 cup chopped red onions

- 1/2 cup crumbled feta cheese

- 1/4 cup chopped fresh parsley

- 2 tablespoons olive oil

- 2 tablespoons lemon juice

- Salt and pepper to taste

Instructions:

1. In a large salad bowl, combine cooked chickpeas, diced cucumbers, diced tomatoes, chopped red onions, crumbled feta cheese, and chopped fresh parsley.

2. In a small bowl, whisk together olive oil, lemon juice, salt, and pepper to make the dressing.

3. Drizzle the dressing over the salad, toss gently to combine, and serve.

Turkey and Avocado Wrap

Ingredients:

• Whole-grain wrap or tortilla

• 4 oz sliced turkey breast

• 1/4 avocado, sliced

• 1/2 cup mixed greens

• 1/4 cup sliced red bell pepper

• 1 tablespoon hummus (optional)

• Olive oil for cooking

Instructions:

1. Lay out the whole-grain wrap or tortilla. Spread a thin layer of hummus (if using) over the wrap.

2. Arrange sliced turkey breast, avocado slices, mixed greens, and sliced red bell pepper on the wrap. Roll up the wrap tightly, tucking in the sides as you go.

3. Slice in half diagonally for easier eating.

Broccoli and Quinoa Salad

Ingredients:

• 2 cups cooked quinoa

• 2 cups steamed broccoli florets

• 1/2 cup diced red bell pepper

• 1/2 cup diced red onion

• 1/4 cup sliced almonds

• 1/4 cup dried cranberries

- 2 tablespoons olive oil

- 2 tablespoons balsamic vinegar

- Salt and pepper to taste

Instructions:

1. In a large bowl, combine cooked quinoa, steamed broccoli florets, diced red bell pepper, diced red onion, sliced almonds, and dried cranberries.

2. In a small bowl, whisk together olive oil, balsamic vinegar, salt, and pepper to make the dressing.

3. Drizzle the dressing over the salad, toss gently to combine, and serve.

Tomato Basil Quinoa Bowl

Ingredients:

- 1 cup cooked quinoa

- 1 cup diced fresh tomatoes

- 1/4 cup chopped fresh basil

- 2 tablespoons grated Parmesan cheese

- 1 tablespoon olive oil

- 1 tablespoon balsamic vinegar

- Salt and pepper to taste

Instructions:

1. In a serving bowl, layer cooked quinoa, diced fresh tomatoes, and chopped fresh basil. Sprinkle grated Parmesan cheese on top.

2. In a small bowl, whisk together olive oil, balsamic vinegar, salt, and pepper to make the dressing.

3. Drizzle the dressing over the quinoa bowl and serve.

Baked Salmon with Lemon and Dill

Ingredients:

• 4 salmon fillets

• 2 lemons, thinly sliced

• 4 sprigs fresh dill

• 2 cloves garlic, minced

• 2 tablespoons olive oil

• Salt and pepper to taste

Instructions:

1. Preheat your oven to 375°F (190°C).

2. Place each salmon fillet on a separate piece of aluminum foil. Season the salmon with minced garlic, olive oil, salt, and pepper.

3. Top each fillet with lemon slices and a sprig of fresh dill. Seal the aluminum foil packets tightly.

4. Bake in the preheated oven for about 15-20 minutes, or until the salmon is cooked through and flakes easily with a fork.

5. Serve hot.

Quinoa and Black Bean Stuffed Peppers

Ingredients:

• 4 bell peppers, any color

• 1 cup cooked quinoa

• 1 cup canned black beans, drained and rinsed

• 1 cup diced tomatoes

• 1/2 cup corn kernels (fresh, frozen, or canned)

• 1/2 cup shredded cheddar cheese

• 1 teaspoon chili powder

• 1/2 teaspoon cumin

• Salt and pepper to taste

• Olive oil for cooking

Instructions:

1. Preheat your oven to 375°F (190°C). Cut the tops off the bell peppers, remove seeds, and rinse them.

2. In a skillet, heat a bit of olive oil over medium heat. Add diced tomatoes and corn kernels. Sauté for about 3-4 minutes until heated through.

3. In a large bowl, combine cooked quinoa, black beans, sautéed tomatoes and corn, shredded cheddar cheese, chili powder, cumin, salt, and pepper.

4. Stuff each bell pepper with the quinoa mixture. Place the stuffed peppers in a baking dish and cover with aluminum foil.

5. Bake for about 30-35 minutes, or until the peppers are tender.

6. Serve hot.

Chicken and Vegetable Stir-Fry

Ingredients:

• 2 boneless, skinless chicken breasts, cut into strips

• 2 cups broccoli florets

- 1 cup sliced bell peppers (assorted colors)

- 1 cup sliced carrots

- 1/2 cup sliced mushrooms

- 2 cloves garlic, minced

- 1/4 cup low-sodium soy sauce

- 2 tablespoons hoisin sauce

- 1 tablespoon sesame oil

- 2 tablespoons olive oil

- Cooked brown rice for serving

Instructions:

1. In a bowl, mix together low-sodium soy sauce, hoisin sauce, and sesame oil. Set aside.

2. In a large skillet or wok, heat olive oil over medium-high heat. Add minced garlic and sauté for about 30 seconds until fragrant.

3. Add chicken strips and stir-fry until they are no longer pink, about 5-6 minutes. Remove from the skillet and set aside.

4. In the same skillet, add a bit more olive oil if needed. Add broccoli florets, sliced bell peppers, sliced carrots, and sliced mushrooms. Stir-fry for about 5 minutes until the vegetables are tender-crisp.

5. Return the cooked chicken to the skillet. Pour the sauce mixture over the chicken and vegetables.

6. Stir-fry for an additional 2-3 minutes until everything is heated through. Serve the chicken and vegetable stir-fry over cooked brown rice.

Lentil and Sweet Potato Soup

Ingredients:

• 1 cup dried green or brown lentils, rinsed and drained

• 2 sweet potatoes, peeled and diced

• 1 onion, chopped

• 2 cloves garlic, minced

- 1 teaspoon ground cumin

- 1/2 teaspoon ground coriander

- 1/4 teaspoon ground turmeric

- 1/4 teaspoon smoked paprika

- 6 cups low-sodium vegetable broth

- 2 tablespoons olive oil

- Salt and pepper to taste

Instructions:

1. In a large pot, heat olive oil over medium heat.

2. Add chopped onions and minced garlic. Sauté for about 3-4 minutes until softened. Add diced sweet potatoes and cook for another 3-4 minutes.

3. Stir in ground cumin, ground coriander, ground turmeric, smoked paprika, salt, and pepper. Cook for an additional minute until fragrant.

4. Add rinsed lentils and vegetable broth to the pot.

5. Bring the mixture to a boil, then reduce heat, cover, and simmer for about 20-25 minutes, or until lentils and sweet potatoes are tender.

6. Serve hot.

Greek Salad with Grilled Shrimp

Ingredients:

• 1-pound large shrimp, peeled and deveined

• 4 cups mixed greens

• 1 cup cherry tomatoes, halved

• 1 cucumber, sliced

• 1/2 cup Kalamata olives, pitted and sliced

• 1/2 cup crumbled feta cheese

• 2 tablespoons olive oil

• 2 tablespoons lemon juice

• 1 teaspoon dried oregano

• Salt and pepper to taste

Instructions:

1. In a bowl, whisk together olive oil, lemon juice, dried oregano, salt, and pepper to make the dressing. Set aside.

2. Season the shrimp with a little olive oil, salt, and pepper. Grill the shrimp for about 2-3 minutes per side, or until they turn pink and opaque.

3. In a large salad bowl, combine mixed greens, cherry tomatoes, cucumber slices, Kalamata olives, and crumbled feta cheese.

4. Add the grilled shrimp on top of the salad.

5. Drizzle the dressing over the salad, toss gently to coat, and serve.

Baked Chicken and Broccoli Casserole

Ingredients:

• 4 boneless, skinless chicken breasts

• 4 cups broccoli florets

- 1 cup cooked quinoa

- 1 cup shredded cheddar cheese

- 1/2 cup low-sodium chicken broth

- 1/4 cup Greek yogurt

- 2 cloves garlic, minced

- 1 teaspoon dried thyme

- Salt and pepper to taste

- Olive oil for cooking

Instructions:

1. Preheat your oven to 375°F (190°C). Season chicken breasts with salt, pepper, and dried thyme.

2. In a large oven-safe skillet, heat olive oil over medium-high heat. Add chicken breasts and sear for 2-3 minutes per side until golden brown. Remove the chicken from the skillet and set aside.

3. In the same skillet, add minced garlic and sauté for about 30 seconds until fragrant. Stir in cooked quinoa, broccoli florets, low-sodium chicken broth, and Greek yogurt.

4. Place the seared chicken breasts on top of the mixture. Sprinkle shredded cheddar cheese over the chicken and mixture.

5. Transfer the skillet to the preheated oven and bake for 20-25 minutes, or until the chicken is cooked through and the casserole is bubbly.

6. Serve hot.

Spinach and Mushroom Stuffed Chicken

Ingredients:

• 4 boneless, skinless chicken breasts

• 2 cups fresh spinach leaves

• 1 cup sliced mushrooms

• 1/2 cup low-sodium chicken broth

• 1/4 cup grated Parmesan cheese

- 2 cloves garlic, minced

- 2 tablespoons olive oil

- Salt and pepper to taste

Instructions:

1. Preheat your oven to 375°F (190°C). Season chicken breasts with salt and pepper.

2. In a skillet, heat olive oil over medium-high heat. Add minced garlic and sauté for about 30 seconds until fragrant. Add sliced mushrooms and cook for 3-4 minutes until they release their moisture.

3. Stir in fresh spinach leaves and cook for another 2-3 minutes until wilted. Remove the skillet from heat and let it cool slightly.

4. In a bowl, combine the cooked spinach and mushroom mixture with grated Parmesan cheese.

5. Slice a pocket into each chicken breast and stuff them with the spinach and mushroom mixture. Place the stuffed chicken

breasts in a baking dish. Pour low-sodium chicken broth over the chicken.

6. Bake in the preheated oven for 25-30 minutes, or until the chicken is cooked through.

7. Serve hot.

Lentil and Vegetable Curry

Ingredients:

• 1 cup dried green or brown lentils, rinsed and drained

• 2 cups mixed vegetables (e.g., bell peppers, peas, carrots)

• 1 small onion, finely chopped

• 2 cloves garlic, minced

• 1 can (14 oz) diced tomatoes

• 1 can (14 oz) light coconut milk

• 2 tablespoons curry powder

• 1 tablespoon olive oil

- Salt and pepper to taste

- Cooked brown rice for serving

Instructions:

1. In a large skillet, heat olive oil over medium heat. Add chopped onion and minced garlic. Sauté for 2-3 minutes until fragrant.

2. Stir in curry powder and cook for an additional minute. Add the mixed vegetables and sauté for another 3-4 minutes.

3. Pour in the diced tomatoes (with their juices), rinsed lentils, and light coconut milk. Stir well.

4. Bring the mixture to a simmer and let it cook for 15-20 minutes, or until the vegetables are tender and the curry has thickened.

5. Season with salt and pepper to taste. Serve the lentil and vegetable curry over cooked brown rice.

Tofu and Broccoli Stir-Fry

Ingredients:

- 1 block (14 oz) extra-firm tofu, cubed

- 4 cups broccoli florets

- 1 bell pepper, thinly sliced

- 1/4 cup low-sodium soy sauce

- 2 tablespoons honey or maple syrup

- 1 tablespoon sesame oil

- 2 cloves garlic, minced

- 1 teaspoon grated ginger

- 2 tablespoons olive oil

- Cooked brown rice for serving

Instructions:

1. In a bowl, whisk together low-sodium soy sauce, honey or maple syrup, sesame oil, minced garlic, and grated ginger to make the sauce. Set aside.

2. In a large skillet, heat olive oil over medium-high heat. Add cubed tofu and cook until golden brown on all sides.

3. Remove tofu from the skillet and set aside.

4. In the same skillet, add a bit more olive oil if needed. Add broccoli florets and sliced bell pepper. Stir-fry for about 4-5 minutes until they are tender-crisp.

5. Return the cooked tofu to the skillet. Pour the sauce over the tofu and vegetables. Stir-fry for an additional 2-3 minutes until everything is heated through.

6. Serve the tofu and broccoli stir-fry over cooked brown rice.

Tomato Basil Zucchini Noodles

Ingredients:

• 4 medium zucchinis, spiralized into noodles

• 2 cups cherry tomatoes, halved

• 1/4 cup fresh basil leaves, torn

• 2 cloves garlic, minced

• 2 tablespoons olive oil

• 1/4 cup grated Parmesan cheese (optional)

• Salt and pepper to taste

Instructions:

1. In a large skillet, heat olive oil over medium heat.

2. Add minced garlic and sauté for about 30 seconds until fragrant. Add spiralized zucchini noodles and cherry tomatoes to the skillet.

3. Sauté for 3-4 minutes until the noodles are tender but still slightly crisp. Stir in torn fresh basil leaves.

4. Season with salt and pepper. Sprinkle with grated Parmesan cheese if desired.

5. Serve hot.

Mediterranean Chickpea Salad with Grilled Chicken

Ingredients:

• 2 boneless, skinless chicken breasts

• 1 can (15 oz) chickpeas, drained and rinsed

• 2 cups diced cucumber

- 1 cup cherry tomatoes, halved

- 1/2 cup diced red onion

- 1/4 cup Kalamata olives, pitted and sliced

- 1/4 cup crumbled feta cheese

- 2 tablespoons olive oil

- 2 tablespoons lemon juice

- 1 teaspoon dried oregano

- Salt and pepper to taste

Instructions:

1. Season chicken breasts with olive oil, dried oregano, salt, and pepper.

2. Grill the chicken for about 6-8 minutes per side or until cooked through.

3. In a large salad bowl, combine chickpeas, diced cucumber, cherry tomatoes, diced red onion, Kalamata olives, and

crumbled feta cheese. Slice the grilled chicken and add it to the salad.

4. In a small bowl, whisk together olive oil and lemon juice to make the dressing.

5. Drizzle the dressing over the salad, toss gently to combine, and serve.

Spinach and White Bean Stuffed Mushrooms

Ingredients:

• 8 large portobello mushrooms, stems removed

• 2 cups fresh spinach leaves, chopped

• 1 can (15 oz) white beans (cannellini or navy beans), drained and rinsed

• 1/2 cup grated Parmesan cheese

• 2 cloves garlic, minced

• 2 tablespoons olive oil

• Salt and pepper to taste

Instructions:

1. Preheat your oven to 375°F (190°C). Place the portobello mushrooms on a baking sheet.

2. In a skillet, heat olive oil over medium heat. Add minced garlic and sauté for about 30 seconds until fragrant. Stir in chopped spinach and cook until wilted.

3. In a bowl, combine chopped spinach, white beans, grated Parmesan cheese, salt, and pepper.

4. Stuff each portobello mushroom with the spinach and white bean mixture.

5. Bake in the preheated oven for about 15-20 minutes, or until the mushrooms are tender and the filling is heated through.

6. Serve hot.

Baked Cod with Lemon and Herbs

Ingredients:

• 4 cod fillets

• Zest and juice of 1 lemon

- 2 tablespoons chopped fresh herbs (e.g., parsley, thyme, dill)

- 2 cloves garlic, minced

- 2 tablespoons olive oil

- Salt and pepper to taste

Instructions:

1. Preheat your oven to 375°F (190°C).

2. In a small bowl, combine lemon zest, lemon juice, chopped fresh herbs, minced garlic, olive oil, salt, and pepper to create the marinade.

3. Place the cod fillets in a baking dish. Pour the marinade over the cod fillets, ensuring they are well coated.

4. Bake in the preheated oven for about 15-20 minutes, or until the fish is opaque and flakes easily with a fork.

5. Serve hot.

Butternut Squash and Chickpea Curry

Ingredients:

- 1 butternut squash, peeled, seeded, and diced

- 1 can (15 oz) chickpeas, drained and rinsed

- 1 onion, chopped

- 2 cloves garlic, minced

- 1 can (14 oz) diced tomatoes

- 1 can (14 oz) light coconut milk

- 2 tablespoons curry powder

- 2 tablespoons olive oil

- Salt and pepper to taste

- Cooked brown rice for serving

Instructions:

1. In a large pot, heat olive oil over medium heat. Add chopped onion and minced garlic. Sauté for 2-3 minutes until softened.

2. Stir in curry powder and cook for an additional minute. Add diced butternut squash, chickpeas, diced tomatoes (with their juices), and light coconut milk. Stir well.

3. Bring the mixture to a simmer and cook for 20-25 minutes, or until the butternut squash is tender. Season with salt and pepper to taste.

4. Serve the butternut squash and chickpea curry over cooked brown rice.

Grilled Vegetable and Quinoa Salad

Ingredients:

• 2 cups cooked quinoa

• 2 zucchinis, sliced lengthwise

• 1 red bell pepper, sliced

• 1 yellow bell pepper, sliced

• 1 red onion, sliced

• 1/4 cup balsamic vinegar

• 2 tablespoons olive oil

• 1 tablespoon honey or maple syrup

• 1 teaspoon dried Italian seasoning

- Salt and pepper to taste

- Fresh basil leaves for garnish (optional)

Instructions:

1. Preheat your grill to medium-high heat.

2. In a bowl, whisk together balsamic vinegar, olive oil, honey or maple syrup, dried Italian seasoning, salt, and pepper to make the dressing. Set aside.

3. Brush the sliced vegetables with a little olive oil and grill them for about 2-3 minutes per side until they have grill marks and are tender.

4. In a large salad bowl, combine cooked quinoa and grilled vegetables.

5. Drizzle the dressing over the salad, toss gently to coat, and garnish with fresh basil leaves if desired.

Tomato Basil Salmon

Ingredients:

- 4 salmon fillets

- 2 cups cherry tomatoes, halved

- 1/4 cup fresh basil leaves, chopped

- 2 cloves garlic, minced

- 2 tablespoons olive oil

- Salt and pepper to taste

Instructions:

1. Preheat your oven to 375°F (190°C).

2. In a bowl, combine cherry tomatoes, chopped fresh basil, minced garlic, olive oil, salt, and pepper.

3. Place each salmon fillet on a separate piece of aluminum foil. Spoon the tomato basil mixture over each salmon fillet.

4. Seal the aluminum foil packets tightly. Bake in the preheated oven for about 15-20 minutes, or until the salmon is cooked through.

5. Serve hot.

Quinoa and Kale Stuffed Bell Peppers

Ingredients:

• 4 bell peppers, any color

• 1 cup cooked quinoa

• 2 cups chopped kale leaves

• 1 can (15 oz) black beans, drained and rinsed

• 1 cup diced tomatoes

• 1/2 cup shredded cheddar cheese

• 1/2 teaspoon chili powder

• 1/2 teaspoon cumin

• Salt and pepper to taste

• Olive oil for cooking

Instructions:

1. Preheat your oven to 375°F (190°C). Cut the tops off the bell peppers, remove seeds, and rinse them.

2. In a skillet, heat olive oil over medium heat. Add chopped kale leaves and sauté for about 2-3 minutes until wilted.

3. In a large bowl, combine cooked quinoa, sautéed kale, black beans, diced tomatoes, shredded cheddar cheese, chili powder, cumin, salt, and pepper.

4. Stuff each bell pepper with the quinoa and kale mixture. Place the stuffed peppers in a baking dish and cover with aluminum foil.

5. Bake for about 30-35 minutes, or until the peppers are tender.

6. Serve hot.

Greek Lemon Chicken

Ingredients:

• 4 boneless, skinless chicken breasts

• Zest and juice of 2 lemons

• 2 cloves garlic, minced

• 2 teaspoons dried oregano

- 2 tablespoons olive oil

- Salt and pepper to taste

Instructions:

1. In a bowl, combine lemon zest, lemon juice, minced garlic, dried oregano, olive oil, salt, and pepper to create the marinade.

2. Season chicken breasts with the marinade mixture.

3. Grill or pan-sear the chicken for about 6-8 minutes per side or until cooked through.

4. Serve hot.

Lentil and Spinach Soup

Ingredients:

- 1 cup dried green or brown lentils, rinsed and drained

- 4 cups vegetable broth

- 2 cups chopped spinach leaves

- 1 onion, chopped

- 2 cloves garlic, minced

- 1 carrot, diced

- 1 celery stalk, diced

- 2 tablespoons olive oil

- 1 teaspoon ground cumin

- Salt and pepper to taste

Instructions:

1. In a large pot, heat olive oil over medium heat.

2. Add chopped onion, minced garlic, diced carrot, and diced celery. Sauté for about 3-4 minutes until softened.

3. Stir in ground cumin and cook for an additional minute. Add rinsed lentils and vegetable broth to the pot.

4. Bring the mixture to a boil, then reduce heat, cover, and simmer for about 20-25 minutes, or until the lentils are tender.

5. Stir in chopped spinach leaves and cook for another 2-3 minutes until wilted. Season with salt and pepper to taste.

6. Serve hot.

Broccoli and Brown Rice Casserole

Ingredients:

- 2 cups cooked brown rice

- 2 cups broccoli florets, steamed

- 1 cup shredded cheddar cheese

- 1/2 cup Greek yogurt

- 2 cloves garlic, minced

- 1 teaspoon dried thyme

- Salt and pepper to taste

Instructions:

1. Preheat your oven to 375°F (190°C).

2. In a large bowl, combine cooked brown rice, steamed broccoli florets, shredded cheddar cheese, Greek yogurt, minced garlic, dried thyme, salt, and pepper.

3. Transfer the mixture to a baking dish.

4. Bake in the preheated oven for about 20-25 minutes, or until the casserole is bubbly and the cheese is melted and golden.

5. Serve hot.

CONCLUSION

In conclusion, the treatment and prevention of osteoporosis are crucial aspects of maintaining strong and healthy bones throughout life. Osteoporosis is a condition that requires proactive measures to prevent its onset and effective strategies for management if diagnosed. By focusing on a comprehensive approach that encompasses lifestyle changes, proper nutrition, exercise, and medical interventions, when necessary, individuals can significantly reduce their risk of osteoporosis and its associated complications.

Remember that osteoporosis is not an inevitable part of aging, and with the right knowledge and actions, it is possible to maintain bone health and enjoy an active and fulfilling life. Regular screenings, early detection, and adherence to treatment plans can make a significant difference in managing osteoporosis.

As you embark on your journey to prevent and treat osteoporosis, always consult with healthcare professionals, including your doctor and a registered dietitian, to create a personalized plan that aligns with your specific needs and health status. Together, with informed decisions and a commitment to a bone-healthy lifestyle, you can build a foundation of strength and resilience, ensuring that your bones support you throughout your lifetime